Why We Get Sick

The Underlying Epidemic Behind Most Chronic Illnesses and Tactics for Resisting Its Impact

SIM HELEN

TABLE OF CONTENTS

INTRODUCTION 7

Why Do You Still Get Sick If Your Immune System Defends You? 7

The Human Immune System: A Powerful Defense 11

The Function of the Immune System in Defending the Body 13

The Complexity of Immune Responses 14

Common Misconceptions 14

PART I: KNOWING THE IMMUNE SYSTEM 17

CHAPTER ONE 19

The Anatomy of the Immune System 19

The Key Components of the Immune System 20

How the Immune System Recognizes Threats 22

Innate and Adaptive Immunity 24

CHAPTER TWO 27

The Immune Response: A Delicate Balance 27

The Role of Inflammation and Fever 28

Autoimmune Diseases and Allergies: When the Immune System Misfires 29

PART II: WHY WE GET SICK 31

CHAPTER THREE 33

Pathogens and Disease: The Culprits 33

Bacteria, Viruses, Fungi, and Parasites 34

How Pathogens Invade the Body 35

The Concept of Contagiousness 38

CHAPTER FOUR 39

Lifestyle Factors and Environmental Influences 39

The Impact of Diet, Exercise, and Sleep on Immunity . 39

PART III: IMMUNITY AND DISEASE PREVENTION 45

CHAPTER FIVE 47

Boosting Your Natural Defenses 47

Immune-Boosting Foods 47

The Importance of Regular Exercise 58

Strategies for Stress Reduction 59

CHAPTER SIX 61

Vaccination: The Power of Prevention 61

How Vaccines Work 61

History and Impact of Vaccines on Public Health 62

The Myths and Concerns of Vaccines 63

PART IV: WHAT TO DO WHEN YOU GET SICK 65

CHAPTER SEVEN 67

Recognizing the Signs of Illness 67

Early Signs of Some Diseases............................. 67

When to Seek Medical Attention 71

Home Remedies and Self-Care.............................. 72

CHAPTER EIGHT 75

The Role of Medical Treatments 75

Antibiotics, Antivirals, and Antifungals 75

How Health Care Providers Support the Immune System

.... 80

The Limitations of Medical Interventions 81

PART V: FUTURE FRONTIERS IN IMMUNOLOGY . 83

CHAPTER NINE.. 85

Cutting-Edge Research and Therapies 85

Immunotherapy and Its Promise in Treating Diseases . 85

Advances in Personalized Medicine 86

Genetic Engineering and Its Potential in Immunity...... 88

CHAPTER TEN 91

7-Day Meal Plan to Boost Your Immunity................... 91

CONCLUSION... 95

Empowering Your Health 95

What You Should Remember 95

A Knowledgeable and Proactive Approach to Health .. 97

Take Charge of Your Well-Being............................... 97

INTRODUCTION

Your body's main line of defense against illnesses and infections is your immune system

Why Do You Still Get Sick If Your Immune System Defends You?

I was eight years old when I developed a strong hatred for diseases. It all began that awful morning when I awoke to discover my mother sobbing and writhing in agony. When I questioned her about the thick white fabric around her neck, she told me it contained an herbal remedy.

She had a severe headache and an awkward heart issue that made it difficult for her to eat. She would throw up at the sight of anything more than a fourth of her usual food intake. For more than two years, she suffered. There would occasionally be brief periods of relief, but the pain would soon return. The only respite in her unrelenting anguish was the short-lived relief provided by painkillers.

My sister wasn't immune to the terrible hold of illness as I got older, though. She experienced excruciating stomach discomfort when she woke up one night, and it lasted for more than three years. She cried out in pain, and I can still clearly remember those tears. She was on a lot of medications, but her relief was never lasting. As the cycle persisted, my other sister who had been assisting in maintaining our family unit became ill as well.

It appeared to be a never-ending nightmare. Nearly all of the members of our family have experienced some sort of health issues. I also gave in to a horrible stomach condition that refused to go away while I was getting ready to start high school. That pain took more than three months to go away. "Why do we get sick?" was the question that had been bothering me for years, and I finally questioned my dad during this experience.

Every time I saw someone confined to a sickbed, I couldn't help but ask myself this one question. My sister had a close friendship with a lady in our neighborhood. She got sick and was taken to the hospital right away. The devastating news of her untimely death broke our hearts.

The terrible death of that lady struck me deeply, and I found myself asking my father the same question: "Why do we get sick?"

As a medical professional, my father received a steady flow of people with various illnesses coming into our home every day. I had made several visits to hospitals, where I saw patients with varying degrees of health and diseases. "Why do we get sick?" remained a burning question. Eventually, after our neighbor passed away tragically and considering my own experiences, I started to question if there is a cure for diseases.

The subject of "Infectious Diseases and the Immune System" was brought up in our biology class one day by my teacher. I started to understand a little bit about the causes of our illnesses in that very classroom. He highlighted a few points, one of which was that our immune system works nonstop to defend and keep us healthy. At this moment, I started thinking about something else "Why do we still fall sick if our immune system is defending us?" When I got home that day, I wanted further explanation, so I told my father about the new subject the teacher introduced to us. He carefully clarified the intricacies of the subject, and I recognized then that the key to solving the challenges of illness prevention and therapy was discovering the causes of our illnesses. That freshly discovered knowledge was the impetus for my research expedition.

The result of my search for answers is this book. You will learn about the hidden epidemics that underlie many chronic illnesses as you read through these pages and gain techniques to mitigate their effects. You can start down the path to a longer, happier, and healthier life with this knowledge. So, I'd like to invite you to come along with me through the pages of this book as we try to figure out the fundamental causes of illness and what we can do about it.

Joining forces, we may conquer the powerful adversaries threatening our health and become champions of energy and health.

Happy reading!

The Human Immune System: A Powerful Defense

The human body is always at battle with massive armies of tiny adversaries. Pathogens, whether they are bacteria, parasites, fungi, or viruses, will utilize all methods necessary to breach the defenses of our systems. They can enter through wounds, the mouth when we swallow, or even as we breathe in.

They make every effort to develop and reproduce once they're inside our bodies, which has negative effects. These bacteria cause a variety of ailments by harming our cells or releasing their toxins, from the common cold and measles to possibly harmful conditions like tuberculosis and malaria.

We are fortunate to have an internal defense mechanism called the immune system that was created to counteract these dangers. Organs, tissues, and cells work together in a complicated network to support this very intricate setup. Its goal, however, is very straightforward: to identify, neutralize, and eliminate invaders while also keeping a record of them in case they come back at a later time.

The immune system has equipped itself with a variety of assault strategies to accomplish this amazing achievement. Some immune system elements engulf and destroy all infections without discrimination. Certain invading species or their harmful by-products can be precisely eliminated by particular proteins produced by other components.

The inventiveness of a lengthy range of scientists and a sequence of breakthroughs that occurred over many decades is largely responsible for our current understanding of how such a complex defense system functions. Because of the work of those scientists, we now have a solid grasp of the immune system's numerous mechanisms for identifying and combating these invaders as well as how it detects the start of an assault.

We are aware of how the immune system avoids harming the body's cells and tissues, but we are also aware of how, regrettably, it occasionally goes wrong and unleashes lethal forces on the same body it is meant to defend.

The Function of the Immune System in Defending the Body

Your body's main line of defense against illnesses and infections is your immune system, which is not simply another organ. It is the superhero of your body, and like any superhero, it possesses a wide range of skills. Invaders of countless varieties may be recognized and remembered by it, and it can also create potent weapons to repel them and even treat any injuries they may have left behind.

Consider your immune system to be a top-tier intelligence service. Immune cells act as agents and patrol your body, looking for invaders and eliminating them.

These agents have memory, so once they've faced an opponent; they never forget how to get the better of it.

You don't continually become sick from the same ailment because of this incredible memory.

The Complexity of Immune Responses

But there's an intriguing twist: the immune system is not just one cohesive mechanism. It's a sophisticated team of cells, proteins, and organs working in unison.

Your immune system organizes a coordinated series of reactions when it finds an invader, each performing a specific function. Invading cells are engulfed by certain cells, while others release specialized proteins called antibodies to identify and destroy them.

Imagine it as a complex game of chess. The immune cells in your body function tactically to protect your general health. Similar to the chess pieces, each immune cell has a specific move and purpose.

Common Misconceptions

The immune system is now surrounded by misconceptions while having amazing capabilities. One popular misunderstanding is that having a robust immune system guarantees you'll never get sick, but that's not accurate.

A strong immune system can nevertheless allow a few invaders to get through, and even the toughest fortress may have a breach. It's not a matter of never becoming sick, but rather of how well your body handles disease when it does.

Your immune system doesn't simply respond to threats it has identified; it also keeps things in check to prevent needless collateral harm

In this book, the immune system's secrets will be revealed, along with the reasons why we still get sick despite its vigilance and, most significantly, what you can do to maintain and enhance this amazing defensive system. By the end of this book, you'll be equipped with the information and skills necessary to make your immune system the primary protector of your health.

Sickness can be uncomfortable and bothersome. Over time, it might potentially result in more severe health issue. Because of this, it's critical to recognize and address the root cause of illness.

PART I: KNOWING THE IMMUNE SYSTEM

<u>*A robust immune system relies on the immune system's exceptional capacity to differentiate between the body's own cells, or self and foreign cells, or nonself.*</u>

CHAPTER ONE

The Anatomy of the Immune System

Every invading microbe, from bacteria to viruses, carries antigens like identification cards. Your immune system's ability to discern these cards is crucial.

The body's immune system consists of individual components that work together to find and destroy bacteria, viruses, and diseases. Each part of the immune system must function in order to detect and differentiate unhealthy organisms from healthy tissues.

Together, each component of the immune system works to keep the person healthy and free from disease, bacteria, viruses, and fungi.

The Key Components of the Immune System

1. Bone Marrow

The primary point of production of the cells of the immune system, bone marrow, is a substance found inside the bones in the hips and thighs. White blood cells, red blood cells, and platelets are found in bone marrow.

2. Thymus

The thymus is the organ in charge of the growth and release of T cells. It is where the T-cells that are critical to the adaptive immune system build self-tolerance before being released into the body's system. The thymus produces a type of white blood cell, the T-cell. It is found just below the chest bone. Lymphocytes and lymphoid tissues constitute the thymus

3. Lymph Nodes

Lymph nodes are part of the lymphatic system, widely distributed throughout the body. They are responsible for trapping foreign particles and filtering pathogens within the body.

4. Spleen

Located in the upper left abdominal section, the spleen is structured similarly to an oversized lymph node and works as a blood filter.

a) Structure: Made up of two distinct parts, the red pulp and white pulp. The spleen keeps the body healthy by removing foreign substances from the blood.

b) Red pulp: Red blood cell filtration, which purges the body of damaged cells, happens here.

c) White pulp: Responsible for immune response, white pulp includes T cells and B cells that fight antigens in the bloodstream for improved health.

5. Mucosa-Associated Lymphoid Tissue (MALT)

The mucosa-associated lymphoid tissue is the major component of lymphatic tissue and is a diffusion system composed of modest quantities of lymphoid tissue situated in the mucosal linings of the body. The MALT protects the body from various antigens and has a differential naming structure that refers to multiple locations of the tissue within the body such as:

Bronchial or Tracheal-Associated Lymphoid Tissue

Nasal Associated Lymphoid Tissue

Gut Associated Lymphoid Tissue

6. Lymphocyte Recirculation

It is the process by which lymphocytes migrate across all of the body's tissues—lymphoid and non-lymphoid—to flush away antigens and protect a person from illness, germs, and viruses.

How the Immune System Recognizes Threats

Imagine a sentry at the gates of a castle, skillfully identifying friend from foe. Similar processes take place within your immune system. To recognize threats, it relies on proteins known as antigens. Antigens are like the faces of intruders – unique and distinctive.

Every invading microbe, from bacteria to viruses, carries antigens like identification cards. Your immune system's ability to discern these cards is crucial. It does so through a sophisticated network of receptors that "read" these antigenic signatures, allowing your body to pinpoint the threat and mount a response.

For example, when you catch a cold, your immune system recognizes the antigens on the surface of the cold virus, quickly mobilizing to eradicate it. This ability to distinguish between self and non-self is a marvel of nature.

Your body's cells have proteins that are antigens- human leukocyte antigens (HLAs). These are on the surface of almost all cells in the human body. HLAs are in large amounts on the surface of white blood cells. They help the immune system differentiate between body tissue and substances that are not from your body. Your immune system becomes used to certain antigens and typically does not respond negatively to them.

Innate and Adaptive Immunity

The immune system possesses a dual nature: innate and adaptive immunity. It's as if it has both a rapid-response SWAT team and a highly trained special ops unit.

The first line of protection for your body is innate immunity. It is the swift, non-specific reaction that acts immediately upon detecting a threat. Think of it as the initial alarms that go off when an intruder enters your home. Innate immunity is your body's way of buying time for the more precise adaptive immune response to gear up.

Examples of innate immunity include:

- Skin
- Cough reflex
- Stomach acid
- Enzymes in tears and skin oils
- Mucus, which traps germs and tiny particles

Innate immunity can help protect us from various pathogens, including the coronavirus that causes COVID-19. Depending on what kind of pathogen, the details and effectiveness of the reaction may vary.

Adaptive Immunity, on the other hand, is tailored to the specific threat. It is like having a detective who carefully analyzes the intruder's identity and develops a precise plan of action. It is why you won't catch the same cold twice – your immune system remembers past encounters and responds more efficiently.

For instance, when you get a vaccine, it triggers an adaptive immune response. Your body learns to recognize and combat the virus or bacteria in question. This is why vaccines are so effective in preventing diseases.

It's common to think of the innate and adaptive immune systems as two distinct, opposing parts of the host defense; however, they often cooperate, with the innate response serving as the primary host defense, after a few days, when antigen-specific T and B cells have undergone clonal proliferation, the adaptive response starts to become more noticeable.

Components of the innate system contribute to the activation of the antigen-specific cells. Also, the antigen-specific cells boost their responses by engaging innate effector techniques to achieve total control over the invading microorganisms. Thus, while the innate and adaptive immune responses are fundamentally different in their mechanisms of action, the synergy between them is essential for an intact, fully effective immune response.

CHAPTER TWO

The Immune Response: A Delicate Balance

For optimum health, it's essential to comprehend the delicate balance of your immune system's reactions.

The primary function of the immune system is to detect pathogens. It involves separating "self" from "non-self" in immunology: Our organs' cells are self, but pathogenic bacteria and viruses are non-self. But what about the countless numbers of bacteria that inhabit our digestive systems and give us advantages like vitamin production and food digestion? Are they an ally or an enemy?

A hazardous kind of intestinal inflammation known as colitis may be activated by an immune system that views our helpful gut flora as an adversary. Equally harmful is an immune system that does nothing while gut microorganisms overstep predetermined boundaries. For a body to operate well, it is essential to comprehend the intricate balance between these two states.

Considering its intricacy, the immune system reacts to threats in diverse ways. It understands when to use force against an opponent and when to negotiate tactfully. For instance, it reacts proportionately to mild injuries. It removes the damaged tissue, restores it and you recover quickly. On the other hand, when it comes across a severe illness, it goes all out, raising the alert through fever and inflammation to ward off the intruder. The ability to tell a friend from an adversary is what maintains the equilibrium.

The Role of Inflammation and Fever

The warning signs and sirens of your body's defensive mechanism include inflammation and fever. The immune system's potency is increased by inflammation, a localized reaction that draws additional immune cells to the area. It is comparable to more troops entering the fight. However, severe or protracted inflammation can cause collateral damage and disorders like chronic inflammation, which is the underlying cause of many diseases.

Contrarily, a fever is your body's approach to increasing the temperature so that some invaders would not survive. Your internal heat is fending off invaders. Also, fever should be managed, much like inflammation. Your body might suffer effects from an abnormally high temperature as much as the infection it is making an attempt to fight.

Autoimmune Diseases and Allergies: When the Immune System Misfires

Things can go wrong occasionally during the intricate functions of the immune system. Autoimmune diseases can develop due to the immune system mistaking your own cells for foreign invaders. An example of the immune system mistaking and targeting healthy tissues includes multiple sclerosis, rheumatoid arthritis, and lupus.

When the immune system overreacts to innocuous elements like pollen or specific foods, it results in allergies.

Your immune system takes on the role of a security guard who is too cautious and looks for danger when there is none.

There may be a variety of unpleasant or even life-threatening responses as a result.

Despite the differences in appearance between hay fever, asthma, eczema, and food allergies, these conditions are all classified as "allergic disorders" because they are developed by the immune system's reaction to innocuous substances like pollen or peanuts.

For optimum health, it's essential to comprehend the delicate balance of your immune system's reactions.

PART II: WHY WE GET SICK

<u>There is a cause for every disease. However, some diseases have symptoms that are so unclear that they are challenging to diagnose. The diseases could be bacterial, viral, malignant, autoimmune, digestive, or STD-related.</u>

CHAPTER THREE

Pathogens and Disease: The Culprits

Pathogens are everywhere in the globe. Experts claim that there exist more viruses on Earth than there are stars in the entire cosmos. A relatively small number of these microorganisms pose a threat to your health. Some of them can even be useful. You can become ill in a number of ways from these infectious agents. The poisons they occasionally release can harm tissue. Sometimes, they trigger an intense immune reaction that causes havoc to both healthy and sick tissue.

This immune response is also a means by which pathogens propagate. They can locate a new host to infect by sneezing, coughing, and diarrhea, to name a few methods. Human actions allowed these infectious agents to proliferate. It's possible to sneeze or cough into your hands before touching objects or other people. Cooking with filthy hands might potentially transmit them to the meal.

In the kitchen, uncooked food can transfer pathogens to other foods. Additionally, after stroking an animal or while changing your child's diaper, you might become infected.

Bacteria, Viruses, Fungi, and Parasites

Four primary kinds of pathogens stand out among the diverse disease-causing agents. Bacteria are a kind of single-celled microorganisms that have a wide range of traits. Others, like the infamous Streptococcus or Staphylococcus, can cause havoc in your body while others, including those that help with digestion, are useful. The smallest troublemakers of them all, viruses, come next.

They need to take over your cells to proliferate since they are protein-coated genetic material. Consider them as microscopic hijackers, and diseases like COVID-19, the common cold, and the flu as their pillaged homeland. Fungi, commonly represented by molds and yeasts, can also be dangerous. Athlete's foot, thrush, and other invasive fungal diseases are caused by them.

Then there are parasites, which can be anything from tiny protozoa to enormous worms. The Plasmodium parasite, which causes malaria, and tapeworm infections are two well-known instances of the damage that parasites may do.

How Pathogens Invade the Body

Pathogens are sly snoopers. In order to get past your body's defenses, they employ a variety of strategies. Bacteria may enter the body through wounds, contaminated food, or respiratory droplets. While parasites can use vectors like mosquitoes to enter the body, viruses frequently do so through respiratory secretions or physical contact. Contrarily, fungi infect people by preying on their compromised immune systems.

Take tuberculosis, for instance. If a person with the infection coughs, tiny airborne particles carrying Mycobacterium tuberculosis are released, entering the body. If you inhale these particles, the bacteria may settle in your lungs and result in the disease.

Host-Cell Invasion: Only organisms outside of cells or on the surface of cells can be detected by the immune system. The system is now exposed to assault from its own cells.

For instance, Shigella flexneri, bacteria that infects individuals through feces-contaminated foods, causing severe diarrhea and vomiting, first clings to and then penetrates macrophages—immune cells that have particular expertise in destroying invading pathogens—as they roam the intestines.

In the host cell, where the immune system is not present, Shigella multiplies unchecked. At some point, the infected macrophage dies and exudes fresh bacteria, which disperse to neighboring epithelial cells and infect them, causing the intestinal tissue to face destruction. If contaminated food enters the intestinal tract, Listeria monocytogenes, bacteria that can cause meningitis and sudden abortion in pregnant women, first attack epithelial cells there.

Once inside the bloodstream, bacteria spread and grow there. The immune cells of the patient are breached in the blood, and the infection is spread throughout the body by the immune cells. Meningitis, a potentially fatal infection of the membrane protecting the brain, may result from those infected cells entering the brain and releasing Listeria. The pathogen can be released into the fetus if the infected cells pass through the placenta of a pregnant woman, and the following infection can harm the unborn child.

As one of the body's natural defenses against contagious microorganisms, the lining of cells on the surface of the intestines or the lungs is another target. The skin, intestines, lungs, and urinary tracts are just a few of the surfaces exposed to the outside. These surfaces are lined by epithelial cells and interwoven so that no virus or bacterium can pass through.

These surfaces also have immune cells covering them that are prepared to combat any alien structure that invades the area. Since these cells are on the inner side of the epithelial barrier, many pathogens first infect them to create a bridgehead from which they can release their offspring into the tissues and blood vessels on the outer side. When this happens, the bloodstream may end up being the route by which they spread throughout the body and infect additional tissues and organs.

Pathogens have developed mechanisms and tactics that allow them to infiltrate host cells. However, the host is frequently actively involved in a pathogen's invasion of a target cell. The plasma membrane, the outer membrane that encircles the host cell, and the coordinated interaction of numerous bacterial and host-cell proteins are required for internalizing pathogens.

The Concept of Contagiousness

The word "contagiousness" evokes both dread and interest. It is the capacity of a pathogen to transmit from person to person. Flu and chickenpox are examples of highly contagious illnesses that can spread like wildfire over a population. In order to stop the spread of a disease, it is essential to understand how contagious it is. Consider COVID-19, a respiratory condition that is extremely contagious. SARS-CoV-2, the virus that causes it, spreads via respiratory droplets released when an infected person coughs, sneezes or speaks. It may also cling to surfaces and spread to people who come into contact with contaminated items.

We have lifted the veil on the disease-causing agents. We can better defend ourselves against these enemies if we understand them.

CHAPTER FOUR

Lifestyle Factors and Environmental Influences

Your choices and the environment you live in significantly impact the health of your immune system, which is greatly affected by the infections it meets. Carefully read as we discuss the crucial impact that lifestyle variables and environmental influences play in determining the tenacity and persistence of your immunological defenses.

The Impact of Diet, Exercise, and Sleep on Immunity

There are several factors that might weaken your immune system, including poor nutrition, insufficient sleep, stress, inactivity, and a disregard for meals high in protein. Your body's defenses depend on these factors for their sustenance.

Diet: Your immune system's fuel source is a well-balanced, nutrient-rich diet. Your immune system's cells require specific nutrients in order to function well, such as vitamins, minerals, and antioxidants found in fruits, vegetables, and whole grains. For instance, white blood cells, the body's immune system's infantry, are produced with the help of vitamin C found in citrus fruits.

A minimum of 10 glasses (2.5 liters of possibly tepid water) of water each day should be consumed in order to maintain optimum hydration.

One of the main things that impact our immune system is an excessive intake of red meat, sugar, fatty foods, and low-fiber diets. These foods cause the body to become inflammatory, which has a negative impact on many bodily functions. Too much sugar consumption reduces the immune system's capacity to fight bacteria.

One of our body's defenses against new and unusual foreign substances continually coming in the form of food is the gut. Compared to other bodily parts, the immune system of the digestive tract encounters the most antigens. Hence, a strong gut is an indication of good health.

DIETS ➤	INCREASE ⬆	DECREASE ⬇
Fruits	Watermelon, berries, apple, citrus fruits (oranges, lemons, Indian gooseberry-Amla), papaya, kiwis	Foods and beverages high in sugar
Vegetables	Coriander, Spinach, Carrots, Mint (Pudina), Tomatoes, Broccoli, Bell Peppers, onions, alternative green vegetables	Fast, packed, or canned food
Proteins and Carbohydrates	Fish, Eggs, Yogurt, Soy, Jaggery and Honey, Whole grains	Processed grains, Read meat.
Nuts	Walnuts, Almonds, Hazelnuts	Highly fried foods
Spices	Ginger, Garlic, Turmeric (Haldi), Cinnamon (Dalchini), Basil (Tulsi), Cumin (Jeera), Black Peppers, Cloves	Alcohol and Soda based drinks
Herbs	Green/Herbal tea, Tinospora (Guduchi), Basil (Tulsi), Glycyrrhiza (Licorice), Ginseng	Caffeinated drinks

Exercise: Your immune system benefits from regular physical activity when carefully done. Immune cells are able to patrol and fight off intruders when you regularly exercise because it helps them circulate throughout your body. Exercise shouldn't be taxing, intense compared to what a person is used to, painful or injurious to the body, or done in an unhealthy environment. In such circumstances, it causes stress, which may have a negative impact on immunity.

When beginning a new workout regimen, gradually increase the intensity and length, conduct appropriate warm-ups and cool-downs, and stop whenever you experience exhaustion or stress. Walking, jogging, and swimming are a few regular physical activities. Indoor activities include stretching, yoga (including breathing exercises like Pranayama), and aerobics, cycling, and walking on a treadmill. Engage in physical activity for at least half an hour daily, five days a week, and practice basic breathing exercises.

Sleep: When you get enough peaceful sleep, your body performs maintenance tasks, healing and reviving your body and mind. Studies have found that a good night's sleep increases the release of molecules that fight inflammation and aid in the defense against infections. Your chance of developing cardiovascular disease and obesity, which can weaken your immune system, rises if you consistently lack sleep. Your circadian rhythms—the regular peaks and valleys of bodily hormones that enable typical everyday function need rest to operate normally. The average duration of sleep that adults need each night is seven to eight hours.

Stress and Its Effects on Immune Function

Avoid letting your hectic and demanding work life affect you. Headaches, anxiety, exhaustion, and irritability are just a few of the physical, emotional, and behavioral effects of excessive stress.

Stress causes the body to generate corticosteroid, also known as cortisol, which lowers the body's ability to fight infections and increases susceptibility. Chronic stress may result in overeating unhealthy foods or alcohol consumption, along with falling immunity and nutritional flaws.

The Role of Environmental Toxins in Disease

Your immune system's health is significantly affected by your external surroundings. The environment is full of pollutants, some of which can seriously compromise your immune system and general health. Take air pollution as an example. Particulate matter and chemical-filled, polluted air can irritate your respiratory system and impair your body's natural immune system in the lungs. You become more vulnerable to illnesses like respiratory infections as a result.

In this chapter, we've explored how your daily decisions—from what you eat to how much sleep you get to how you handle stress—intersect to affect the health and responsiveness of your immune system. You may promote your immune system's health and strengthen your body's defenses against disease by taking proactive measures upon the discovery you have made.

PART III: IMMUNITY AND DISEASE PREVENTION

<u>*You will experience frequent bouts of illness if your immune system is weak.*</u>

CHAPTER FIVE

Boosting Your Natural Defenses

Now that you know the effects environmental circumstances and lifestyle choices have on your immune system, it is crucial to uncover some proactive measures you can take to strengthen your body's defenses.

Immune-Boosting Foods

You may think of some foods as your immune system's collaborators since they give it the vital support required to work at its best. The finest meals that offer this support are those in a balanced diet. Your immune system can be maintained by eating foods high in protein, vitamin A, vitamin C, vitamin E, iron, and zinc. The foods that naturally contain lots of these nutrients will be the best for boosting your body's defenses. Such foods include:

1. Citrus Fruits

Oranges and grapefruits are examples of citrus fruits that are rich in vitamin C, which is believed to help the immune system. Men should take 90 mg of vitamin C daily, while adult women should take 75 mg. Vitamin C supports the immune system by assisting the body in tissue repair and preserving the health of blood vessels and the skin. Additionally, vitamin C is a crucial antioxidant, a compound that enhances immune performance and prevents cell aging.

2. Blueberries

A recent study demonstrated that specific components of these delectable berries can protect our respiratory tract from infections. These substances are recognized for their antioxidant effects and are referred to as bioflavonoids. They are by-products of plant metabolism. In addition to being a delicious breakfast food, blueberries make a wholesome dessert and a between-meal snack. In delicious and eye-catching quinoa salad, for instance, it can be consumed as lunch.

3. Elderberries

Since the extracts from the black elderberry bush's fruits have anti-inflammatory effects and are abundant in flavonoids, which are known to protect our lungs, the fruits have long been utilized in syrups and lozenges.

Elderberry syrup is a widely used treatment for the flu, the common cold, and sinus infections.

4. Watermelon

You might find it interesting to learn that watermelon, one of your favorite summertime treats is a better immune system booster than you previously thought. The vitamins A, B6, and C, along with potassium, are all found in abundance in watermelons. Your body needs all these nutrients to stay healthy as it defends itself from harmful intruders. Also, it offers glutathione, a crucial antioxidant that protects your body from the effects of free radicals, heavy metals, and peroxides - molecules that can harm your cells and make you sick.

5. Papaya

Papaya is one of the best meals for boosting your immune system because it is both delicious and healthful. In addition to having vitamin A, it is the ideal source of vitamin C. Both of these nutrients are essential for the healthy operation of our body's natural defense mechanism, which helps to shield us against infections such as the flu and other illnesses.

6. Kiwi

Kiwis are rich in vitamin C as well as other necessary minerals like vitamin K, potassium, and folate, just like papayas are. The daily intake of vitamin C is virtually tripled in one cup of this delectable fruit. Get it and add it to a fruit salad or smoothie.

7. Tomatoes

Tomatoes have a wealth of vitamin C, just like more common fruits. They also supply us with other important antioxidants, including beta-carotene (which our bodies convert into vitamin A, which is necessary for healthy skin and vision) and vitamin E (which shields cells from damage). According to research, the chemical lycopene, which gives these delectable fruits their red color, is actually considerably increased in tomatoes when they are cooked. Lycopene is a potent antioxidant. It implies that a great Bolognese sauce will also boost your immunity. Just remember to occasionally add sliced tomatoes to a fresh salad or sandwich for an excellent additional source of vitamin C.

8. Spinach

Spinach is a must-have on any list of immune-boosting foods. It has all the elements required to maintain our immune system functioning at its peak, including fiber, vitamins A and C, magnesium, and folate (which aids in cell function and the formation of red blood cells). The best way to enjoy spinach is to eat it raw, so why not add some to your sandwich? It tastes amazing. To retain as many nutrients as possible, if you must cook it, cook it briefly.

9. Sweet Potato

Beta-carotene, which your body converts into vitamin A to fight free radicals, may be found in abundance in sweet potatoes. Doing so will not only enable your immune system to function properly but also slow down the aging process, maintaining the health of your skin and shielding it from ultraviolet (UV) rays. You can obtain about one-third of your recommended daily dose of vitamin C and enough vitamin A for the entire day with just one medium-sized sweet potato. The best part is that such a serving has 100 calories and is free of fat and cholesterol, boosting your immune system without worrying about gaining weight.

10. Broccoli

Broccoli is another great candidate for the title of finest all-around immunity superhero, continuing the list of heroes with immunity. This vegetable is one of the best options for boosting your immune system because it is rich in antioxidants, vitamins A, C, and E, fiber, and slow-digesting-helping fiber.

You may be missing if you haven't prepared broccoli as a snack or side dish. However, be cautious not to overcook this nutrient powerhouse. Instead, delicately steam it until it becomes softer and is ready to be consumed. And feel free to enjoy it raw if you don't mind going a little harder.

11. Garlic

Garlic has long been praised for its health advantages, with claims that it helps prevent heart disease, lower cholesterol, and treat colds and the flu. Allicin, a substance released when garlic is chopped or crushed, is the source of all the health benefits associated with garlic. The antioxidants and allicin in garlic support the immune system and aid in the battle against illness. Garlic will lessen cold symptoms since it has antiviral characteristics, which will help you recover more quickly.

12. Ginger

Numerous bioactive substances found in ginger, such as gingerol, have the potential to exert potent anti-inflammatory and antioxidant effects. Furthermore, it possesses antimicrobial characteristics that can aid in the treatment of infectious diseases.

13. Red Bell Peppers

Because they include vitamins A, and C, beta carotene, and other antioxidants, red bell peppers are beneficial for the immune system. Antioxidants and significant therapeutic properties are provided by vitamin C. Vitamin A, which guards against infections, is produced by the body with the aid of beta-carotene.

14. Oily fish

Omega-3 fatty acids can be found in large quantities in oily fish like salmon, tuna, and pilchards. Research suggests that regular consumption of omega-3 fatty acids may lower the incidence of rheumatoid arthritis (RA).

When the immune system unintentionally targets a healthy bodily part, it can lead to RA, a chronic autoimmune disease. Omega-3 fatty acids assist in reducing the risk of such problems or their symptoms.

15. Chicken

Chicken soup is on the list of meals that are known to strengthen the immune system. You'll recover from a cold or the flu faster and experience fewer side effects as a result. The key to its effectiveness is a combination of substances that inhibit mucus production, which is triggered by white blood cells when a cold virus invades our upper respiratory tract. Experts even assert that your body's defense against the flu is provided by a specific compound called carnosine.

16. Oysters

Oysters are one of the riches of the ocean that we just must include in this list of superfoods. They give the body a rich dosage of nutrients that are crucial for maintaining the immune system's peak performance because they are packed with selenium, iron, vitamins A and C, a lot of protein, and zinc.

Vitamins and minerals typically receive the most attention when discussing immunity, but there are some more frequently underrated heroes that merit recognition. The ability of our immune cells to work properly is ensured by one of these nutrients, zinc. Along with oysters, crabs, lobsters, and mussels also contain it. Nevertheless, exercise caution, as consuming more zinc than the daily suggested amount of 10 milligrams can damage your immune system.

17. Almonds

Almonds are a good source of vitamin E, a potent antioxidant that guards against the harm that free radicals do to cells. Protein and iron, which are two nutrients necessary for a healthy immune system, are also included in almonds. They are simple to locate in any grocery store, ideal as a nutritious snack, and can be included in salads, yogurt, and other dishes.

Almonds should be soaked in water before eating to improve the digestion of the soluble vitamins. Almonds or anything else we soak gets easier to chew and easier for the digestive system to process. But do not remove the skin because it is fiber-rich.

18. Eggs

Few people would include eggs among the meals that support the immune system. Vitamin D, another essential component in regulating and strengthening your immune system response by avoiding upper respiratory tract infections, is abundant in eggs, especially yolks. Roasted or grilled mushrooms can be included in some scrambled eggs or an omelet. Your immune system will benefit even more from these because they are rich in zinc, selenium, and B vitamins.

19. Sunflower Seeds

Vitamin E content in sunflower seeds is high. Furthermore, vitamin E appears to be particularly effective in addressing immune system dysfunction brought on by aging.

20. Walnuts

Walnuts are a good source of vitamin E, and a strong antioxidant, just like almonds and sunflower seeds are. Walnuts are also a good source of folate and riboflavin.

21. Yogurt

Your bones and skin can stay healthy by consuming yogurt, a fantastic source of protein. Infections are initially resisted by healthy tissues. In good health, your skin deters pathogenic organisms like viruses or bacteria. The majority of yogurts contain live cultures, which are bacteria that enhance the health of your gut microbiota in addition to protein. Choosing plain, unsweetened yogurt and including nuts, berries, and a tiny bit of honey in your yogurt will help it remain healthy.

22. Turmeric

Curcumin, the turmeric's key ingredient, has anti-inflammatory and antioxidant properties. Preliminary studies have also demonstrated that curcumin can reduce the activation of B and T cells, macrophages, natural killer cells, and other immune system cells when consumed at moderate levels.

The Importance of Regular Exercise

Weight loss and muscular growth are the two main advantages of exercise for the majority of people.

The advantages of it, however, go beyond the obvious. The immune system and general well-being can both benefit from regular exercise, according to studies. There are numerous hypotheses regarding how exercise strengthens the immune system, and it's likely that this occurs in a number of distinct ways.

In addition to increasing blood flow and clearing bacteria from your lungs, exercise can also reduce stress hormones, create a temporary rise in body temperature that may be protective, and boost antibodies to help fight infections. Immune cells become more efficient as a result of it.

The immune system functions better when you exercise regularly because it decreases inflammation. While short-lived inflammation in reaction to an injury is a normal component of a functioning immune system, long-term inflammation can compromise immunological function.

Spread out your workouts and go slowly. Work your way up to completing a target of 30 minutes by beginning with two 15-minute sessions per day. To measure your progress and recognize your accomplishments, think about maintaining an exercise journal. To maintain your pace, use upbeat music. Above all, remember to have fun.

Strategies for Stress Reduction

Because of the close ties between mind and body, stress can have a negative impact on immunological function if it is not well managed. Utilizing stress reduction strategies can help keep your immune system in good shape:

Mindfulness and Meditation: These techniques can assist in reducing stress hormones and calming the mind.

Yoga: Yoga is a great method for reducing stress because it combines exercise with breathing and relaxation techniques.

Breathing Exercises: Exercises involving deep breathing can cause the body to go into relaxation mode, which lessens the effects of stress.

Social Connection: Having supportive social networks can ease stress and offer emotional support.

You've received concrete advice on how to strengthen your immune system in this chapter, from choosing immune-boosting foods to committing to regular exercise and implementing stress management techniques. You'll be actively supporting your body's natural defenses and ensuring a strong immune response when necessary if you incorporate these routines into your daily life.

CHAPTER SIX

Vaccination: The Power of Prevention

Vaccination is a scientific achievement that humanity has used as a shield to defend itself against numerous terrible diseases. Let's quickly explore the fascinating world of vaccines, debunking common myths while examining how they function and their historical context.

How Vaccines Work

A vaccine is a drug that primes the immune system of the body to fight a disease it has never seen before. Instead of treating an existing sickness, vaccines prevent diseases.

The mechanism by which vaccines function is to train your body to identify particular harmful microorganisms so that your immune system is ready to combat that infection in the future. Vaccines impart us with tiny fragments of diseased or dead microorganisms known as antigens. Although they don't actually cause illness, these antigens act to start the body's immunological response.

The most effective defense against life-threatening infections is immunization (vaccination). Lifelong immunity is provided by some immunizations, and at other times, "catch-up" or "booster" shots are required.

History and Impact of Vaccines on Public Health

Vaccines are nothing new. It all started with the purposeful exposure to cowpox to stop the spread of smallpox in Europe and smallpox vaccinations in China centuries ago. Modern vaccinations were built on the principles of these procedures. Edward Jenner's creation of the smallpox vaccine in the late 18th century was one of the turning points in the history of vaccines.

A demonstration of the effectiveness of immunizations is the 1980 smallpox eradication. Vaccines today shield us from illnesses, including measles, polio, influenza, and COVID-19. They have not only prevented innumerable deaths but also lessened the impact of disease, enabling society to advance.

The Myths and Concerns of Vaccines

Despite their astounding success, vaccines are not free of misunderstandings and worries. In order to retain public confidence and achieve extensive vaccination coverage, it is crucial to dispel these myths and address real concerns.

Some of the misunderstandings include worries about the components of vaccines, the notion that vaccines cause autism (a claim refuted by substantial study), and the idea that vaccination is inferior to spontaneous infection. It's imperative to dispel these misconceptions with solid evidence.

Fear of adverse effects can also be a factor in vaccine apprehension. It is crucial to recognize that vaccinations, like any medical procedure, can have adverse effects, but usually minor and transient. The advantages of vaccination surpass the dangers by averting serious illness and preserving public health.

You have probably already seen the science underpinning vaccines, their historical context, and the fact-based responses to common worries and falsehoods. We can protect our health and the well-being of our communities by making intelligent choices of recognizing the effectiveness of vaccination as a means of prevention.

PART IV: WHAT TO DO WHEN YOU GET SICK

CHAPTER SEVEN

Recognizing the Signs of Illness

Even though illness might come on unexpectedly, recognizing the early warning signs, when to seek medical help, and the best self-care techniques can all make a big difference in your overall health.

Early Signs of Some Diseases

The difference between life and death may depend on one's ability to recognize warning signs and what to seek. Here are some conditions and their warning symptoms:

Cold and Flu: Fever, headaches, more severe pain and exhaustion, and a more persistent, frequently dry cough are just a few of the flu's symptoms. Sneezing, coughing, a sore throat, and a runny or stuffy nose are all signs of a cold. Another possible symptom is a bad temperature, along with a minor headache and body aches.

Eating or weight Conditions: Dehydration, intense thirst, excessive hunger, unintended weight loss, overindulging in food, throwing up, starvation, having a skewed perception of one's physique, obsessive activity, despair, and an excessive intake of laxatives or diet pills.

Skin problems: Skin moles changes, hotness and redness of the face and neck, jaundice, prolonged skin lesions, new skin growths or moles, and thick, red skin with silvery patches are all signs of skin problems.

Heart attack: Long-lasting pain, pressure, squeezing, or a sense of fullness in the middle of the chest; pain or discomfort in other parts of the body, shortness of breath, cold sweats, vertigo, or nausea.

Digestive or stomach problems: Gastrointestinal infections may manifest as blood in the stool or black stools, rectal bleeding, altered bowel habits or an inability to control bowel movements, diarrhea, constipation, vomiting, heartburn, or acid reflux.

Stroke: Arm weakness; face drooping, speech difficulties, quickly escalating dizziness or balance, loss of vision, sudden numbness or weakness, a strong headache or confusion.

Reproductive health conditions: Flow or spotting between periods, genital itchiness, burning, pain or discomfort during intimacy, painful or excessive menstrual flow, excruciating pelvic or abdominal pain, abnormal genital discharge, a feeling of heaviness in the belly area, and frequent urination or urgency in urination.

Emotional problems: Anxiety, despair, tenseness, exhaustion, nightmares and flashbacks, boredom with daily activities, delusions. When you experience extraordinary fatigue or lack of energy, your body may be defending itself from an invader.

Lung problems: Bleeding when coughing, breathing difficulties, a persistent cough, wheezing, pneumonia, or recurrent bronchitis. These signs frequently point to respiratory infections.

Bladder problems: urinary symptoms such as painful or frequent urination, trouble with bladder regulation, blood stains in urine, frequent nighttime urination, wetting the bed, or urine leakage.

Joint or muscle issues: Long-lasting aches and pains in the muscles and body, such as numbness; discomfort, soreness, stiffness, edema, inflammation, or redness around joints; and reduced range of movement or loss of function across all joints or muscles.

Breast problems: Breast or nipple alterations, nipple discharge, strange breast discomfort or soreness, or a thickening or lump in or around the breast or under the arm.

AN OBSERVATION ON CANCER

Many of the warning signals mentioned above can be connected to cancer, as you may have seen if you read carefully. But it's crucial to realize that a single symptom generally does not indicate malignancy. In contrast to one or two symptoms, cancer typically causes a plethora of symptoms. In no case should you attempt to self-diagnose by googling your symptoms. If your symptoms are severe enough, visit a medical practitioner.

A symptom in one area of the body may occasionally indicate a condition in another area. Additionally, symptoms that are unrelated to one another yet are modest on their own may be early indicators of a more serious medical condition or disease. Observe your body, make a list of all your symptoms, and discuss them fully with your doctor.

When to Seek Medical Attention

For prompt and effective care, it's essential to know when to seek medical help. Even though many mild illnesses may be treated at home, some circumstances necessitate the knowledge of a doctor. One or more essential indicators are:

High Fever: Contact a healthcare practitioner if you have a high fever that doesn't go down, especially if it's in a youngster.

Breathing Difficulties: Any chest pain, breathing difficulties, or blue lips or face should be treated promptly.

Severe Symptoms: A healthcare provider should be consulted if your symptoms are severe, ongoing, or getting worse.

Dehydration: Medical attention is needed if you show signs of dehydration including black urine and intense thirst.

Chronic Conditions: Make an early appointment with a healthcare practitioner if you have an underlying medical condition such as diabetes, heart disease, or a compromised immune system.

Extended Illness: It's time to consult a doctor if your condition doesn't get better after a few days or if it lasts for weeks.

Home Remedies and Self-Care

A lot of the time, taking care of yourself at home can help you handle minor diseases and discomfort. However, it's crucial to use these remedies appropriately and never in place of qualified medical attention when necessary.

Nutritious Diet: You may boost your body's defenses by eating healthy foods.

Hydration: Stay hydrated by drinking lots of fluids, especially if you're vomiting, have diarrhea, or have a fever.

Rest: To ward against infections, your body requires energy. It's crucial to rest.

Steam Inhalation: This can alleviate breathing problems and clear up congestion.

OTC Medications: For minor symptoms, over-the-counter medications can be helpful. It is the practice of choosing and using medications responsibly and safely to address ailments or symptoms that one has identified. Acetaminophen and ibuprofen, both available over the counter, are effective painkillers and fever reducers.

Lozenges and Cough Drops: These can relieve coughing and ease sore throats.

Isolation: If you are contagious, take measures to stop other people from getting sick from you.

You should prioritize your health and pay attention to what is happening in your body now that you are aware of the signs to look for. Early diagnosis and treatment can greatly improve the prognosis of a serious illness. So every time a small issue arises, there is no need to freak out, simply pay attention to your body, and if there is a problem, visit a doctor.

You can take charge of your health if you are aware of the early symptoms of sickness, know when to seek medical attention, and know how to take care of yourself at home. This information is essential for providing prompt treatment and a less difficult recovery process.

CHAPTER EIGHT

The Role of Medical Treatments

Let's discuss the crucial role that medical treatments play in assisting your body's immune response as we navigate the complexities of immune defense and sickness. We'll discuss the usage of antibiotics, antivirals, and antifungals, how medical personnel support the immune system, and the significant drawbacks of these therapies.

Antibiotics, Antivirals, and Antifungals

In the fight against infections, these three groups of drugs are formidable allies designed to fight off some infections.

ANTIBIOTICS

Antibiotics are drugs that aid in the treatment of bacterial illnesses. They accomplish this by either eliminating the germs or preventing them from proliferating or replicating. Antibiotic translates to "against life." In theory, an antibiotic is any medication that destroys bacteria within your body.

Many people have lost their lives to common bacterial diseases like strep throat before the discovery of antibiotics in the 1920s. Also, surgery was riskier. Then, life expectancy rose, surgeries became safer, and formerly fatal diseases could be treated after the development of antibiotics in the 1940s. Among the common antibiotics are doxycycline, amoxicillin, and penicillin. Antibiotics are effective in treating the following kinds of infections:

- Strep throat
- Skin infections
- Whooping cough
- Dental infections
- Bacterial pneumonia
- Clostridioides difficile
- Kidney and Bladder infections
- Some sinus and ear infections
- Meningitis (enlargement of the spinal cord and brain)

Antibiotics can only treat bacterial infections. Viruses are the source of most coughs, stomach flu, bronchitis infections, common colds, and sore throats.

They cannot be treated with antibiotics. Sometimes, it's difficult to tell if an infection is bacterial or viral. Before selecting the course of treatment for you, your doctor might request tests. Certain antibiotics are effective against a wide variety of microorganisms. We refer to them as "broad-spectrum." Others target particular germs. They are known as "narrow-spectrum."

ANTIVIRALS

Antiviral medications are a particular kind of medication used to treat viral infections. They work by either eradicating viruses or stopping their proliferation. They either aid the immune system in identifying and eliminating viral intruders or prevent the virus from replicating. Oseltamivir for influenza and acyclovir for herpes infections are two well-known antiviral drugs. A review published in Clinical Microbiology states that over 90 antivirals have been created and are now being used. Antivirals can target any of these viral illnesses:

- HIV infections
- Herpes virus infections
- Influenza virus infections

- Human cytomegalovirus infections
- Varicella-zoster virus infections
- Hepatitis B virus infections
- Hepatitis C virus infections
- Infections with respiratory syncytial viruses
- Human papillomavirus infections resulting in external anogenital warts

ANTIFUNGALS

Fungal infections, which typically affect your skin, hair, and nails, are treated with antifungal medications. Treatment may be required for some fungal infections that develop inside the body. In cases where your immune system is compromised, you are more likely to get a more serious fungal infection. Certain antifungal medications require a prescription. However, your pharmacy sells some over-the-counter.

If you suspect a fungal infection, see your Doctor or Pharmacist. They'll advise you on the antifungal medication to take. Antifungal drugs can be administered as injections, liquids, tablets, ointments, creams, gels, sprays, and suppositories for the genitals.

For information relevant to the antifungal medication you are taking, see the patient information booklet included with your order. Drugs such as nystatin and fluconazole are used to treat different types of fungal infections. The common fungal infections that can be treated with antifungals include:

- Ringworm
- Athlete's foot
- Menstrual thrush
- Fungal nail infection
- Some kinds of severe dandruff

Antifungal medications go by several common names, such as:

- Econazole
- Miconazole
- Fluconazole
- Terbinafine
- Ketoconazole
- Clotrimazole
- Amphotericin

Their mechanism of action involves either eliminating the fungus cells or stopping their growth and division. You should check with your doctor if antifungal drugs are suitable for you, especially:

- If you have any allergies
- If you're using any other medication
- If you have any health issues currently
- If you're pregnant, planning to get pregnant, or are already nursing

It is unsafe to take several antifungal medications while pregnant or nursing. Follow your doctor's or pharmacist's instructions when using antifungal drugs. There is additional usage guidance in the information leaflet that comes with your medication.

How Health Care Providers Support the Immune System

When your immune system is dealing with an infection, medical specialists are essential in helping it. They employ multiple strategies to accomplish this:

Diagnosis: Identifying the causing pathogen aids in choosing the best course of action.

Writing Drug Prescriptions: The right antibiotic, antiviral, or antifungal medication to treat a particular infection can be prescribed by a medical professional, based on the diagnosis.

Healthcare support: Treatment for certain conditions may include supportive measures to help the immune system concentrate on the infection, such as rest, pain management, and hydration.

Immunizations: To prevent infections in the future, medical practitioners administer vaccines to prime the immune system to recognize and defend against particular microorganisms.

The Limitations of Medical Interventions

Notwithstanding their effectiveness, these medical interventions have certain drawbacks. Say for example:

Resistance to Antibiotics: Antibiotic-resistant microorganisms have emerged due to antibiotic overuse and misuse, making some therapies ineffectual.

Resistance to Antivirals: Overusing antivirals can result in the emergence of resistant virus strains, just like overusing antibiotics.

Resistance to Antifungal: Antifungal drugs can also cause fungi to become resistant to them.

Viral Challenges: Certain viruses, such as HIV and the common cold, can evolve quickly, making them extremely difficult to cure.

Side Effects: Negative effects are a part of every medical treatment. Therefore, it's crucial to carefully consider the advantages of using them against the risks.

The best way to guarantee your well-being is to adopt a well-rounded strategy that blends medical interventions with a healthy lifestyle.

PART V: FUTURE FRONTIERS IN IMMUNOLOGY

Nowadays, researchers can generate specialized immune cells, antibodies, and lymphokines in large quantities from immune cell secretions. In addition to revolutionizing immune system research, easy access to these materials has had a profound effect on industry, agriculture, and medicine.

CHAPTER NINE

Cutting-Edge Research and Therapies

As we go more into the field of immunological health, it's crucial that we examine cutting-edge medical research, where innovative treatments and research have the potential to revolutionize how we comprehend and treat illnesses. We will explore the intriguing advancements in immunotherapy, personalized medicine, and the possibility of genetic engineering to improve immune responses.

Immunotherapy and Its Promise in Treating Diseases

By using the body's natural defenses against illness, immunotherapy is a cutting-edge field of study. How we treat diseases like cancer, autoimmune diseases, and allergies has changed significantly because of it. Here's how it functions:

Cancer Immunotherapy

There are cancer cells that evade the immune system's recognition. Checkpoint inhibitors, for example, are immunotherapy medications that aid the immune system's ability to identify and combat cancerous cells. When treating different types of cancer, this method has demonstrated impressive results.

Autoimmune Disease Management

Immunotherapies can prevent autoimmune responses by focusing on particular immune system components. For people suffering from illnesses like multiple sclerosis and rheumatoid arthritis, this method offers hope.

Allergy Desensitization

For those with severe allergies, immunotherapy can help relieve symptoms by gradually desensitizing the immune system to allergens.

Advances in Personalized Medicine

Personalized medicine depends on the fact that no two people are precisely alike. With this method, medical care is customized to each person's genetic composition, way of life, and surroundings. Notable features consist of:

Genetic Testing

Medical professionals may now detect genetic markers that can predispose a person to a particular disease or predict how they will respond to treatment due to advancements in genetics.

Precision Medicine

By using genetic information, medical professionals can reduce trial and error by recommending medicines and treatments most likely to succeed.

Targeted Therapies

Personalized medicine has the capability to identify the genetic alterations responsible for diseases such as cancer and develop targeted therapeutics for those mutations.

Genetic Engineering and Its Potential in Immunity

A key component of contemporary biotechnology is genetic engineering. Utilizing methods like recombinant DNA technology, polymerase chain reaction (PCR), and gene cloning, scientists can modify and amplify particular genes, opening up a wide range of potential uses.

Throughout history, infectious diseases have afflicted humanity, resulting in great misery and presenting substantial obstacles to public health. However, a new era of creativity and optimism has arrived in the fight against infectious illnesses with the development of genetic engineering. We might adopt a totally different strategy for treating and avoiding infectious diseases through genetic engineering, a cutting-edge technology that modifies organisms' DNA.

Genetic engineering has completely changed the development of vaccines, which have been a key component in the fight against infectious diseases. The immune response to traditional vaccines was frequently elicited by organisms that had been weakened or inactivated. Scientists may now produce recombinant vaccines through genetic engineering, wherein infectious genes are introduced into healthy organisms to target an immune response without harming the host. This strategy has sped up the creation of vaccinations against serious viruses such as human papillomavirus (HPV), hepatitis B, and the new coronavirus that causes COVID-19.

Now that it is possible to modify the DNA of pathogens, researchers can reduce or perhaps completely eradicate the pathogens' capacity to cause harm. Scientists can decrease a virus or bacteria's pathogenicity by altering its genetic material, hindering the organisms' capacity to proliferate and propagate.

An enormous risk to public health has arisen from the emergence of germs that are resistant to antibiotics. It is possible to produce new antibiotics through genetic engineering, which presents a viable approach. Scientists have the ability to specifically target and eliminate antibiotic-resistant bacteria using bacteriophages, which are viruses that infect bacteria. They can also create antimicrobial peptides with a reduced risk of resistance development and increased activity against infectious agents.

It is also possible to improve the body's natural defenses against pathogenic infections through genetic engineering. Researchers can increase immune cells' capacity to identify and eradicate infectious agents by introducing particular genes through gene therapy techniques. This strategy, which boosts the immune system's capacity to inhibit viral replication, promises the treatment of persistent viral diseases like HIV.

Accurate and quick diagnostic techniques for infectious diseases are possible by genetic engineering. Early and accurate detection of pathogens is made possible by a PCR (polymerase chain reaction), which amplifies specific genetic material.

Future developments in immunotherapy, personalized medicine, and genetic engineering have the potential to revolutionize illness prevention, diagnosis, and treatment. Good news for anyone seeking better health and well-being: tailored, highly effective treatments that leverage the power of our immune system is possible.

CHAPTER TEN

7-Day Meal Plan to Boost Your Immunity

This plan combines different immune-boosting ingredients to provide a balanced and flavorful diet.

DAY 1

Breakfast: Greek yogurt combined with a honey-glazed citrus salad (kiwi, orange, and grapefruit)

Lunch: Spinach salad dressed with citrus vinaigrette and grilled chicken.

Snack: A glass of watermelon smoothie and some almonds.

Dinner: Steamed broccoli, roasted sweet potatoes, and baked salmon.

DAY 2

Breakfast: Yogurt parfait with berries (strawberries and blueberries).

Lunch: Whole-grain bread served beside a spinach and tomato frittata.

Snack: Slices of papaya tossed with little lemon juice.

Dinner: Mix vegetables and quinoa with grilled chicken.

DAY 3

Breakfast: Yogurt scoop served with a green smoothie (spinach, kiwi, and banana)

Lunch: Whole-grain crackers with tomato and garlic soup.

Snack: Red bell pepper sticks and Carrot served with hummus.

Dinner: Baked cod served over quinoa and broccoli.

DAY 4

Breakfast: Omelet with tomatoes and sautéed spinach.

Lunch: Ginger-turmeric dressing on the surface of spinach and sweet potatoes.

Snack: A blend of walnuts and sunflower seeds.

Dinner: Stir-fried tofu with red bell peppers, broccoli, and a sauce flavored with turmeric.

DAY 5

Breakfast: A touch of honey on a smoothie made with papaya and kiwi.

Lunch: Grilled chicken, spinach, and tomato salad with a citrus dressing.

Snack: Yogurt in a little bowl with minced almonds and honey drizzled over it.

Dinner: Roasted sweet potatoes served with baked salmon and steamed broccoli.

DAY 6

Breakfast: Tomatoes and sautéed spinach with scrambled eggs.

Lunch: Soup made with tomatoes and garlic with wholegrain crackers on the side.

Snack: Blueberries mixed with almonds.

Dinner: Steamed broccoli with a side of quinoa, served with grilled oily fish, such as mackerel.

DAY 7

Breakfast: Orange slices and sunflower seeds garnished with Greek yogurt.

Lunch: Spinach and sweet potato salad with grilled chicken and a ginger-turmeric dressing.

Snack: Carrot sticks and red bell peppers with hummus.

Dinner: Baked chicken breast served with mixed vegetables and quinoa on the side.

Drink plenty of water to stay hydrated throughout the week, and think about indulging in herbal teas that contain immune-stimulating herbs like ginger and echinacea. This meal plan offers a balanced and nutrient-dense diet to strengthen your immune system, incorporating foods that increase immunity.

CONCLUSION

Empowering Your Health

As we reach the end of this exploration - what causes illnesses and the methods to deal with them, the necessity of taking control of your own well-being, and the significance of having an informed and proactive approach to health are important issues to consider.

Throughout this journey, we've learned about the complex functions of the immune system and how much it affects your health, from its defense against sickness to its capacity to recognize and remember foreign invaders. We have covered the importance of lifestyle choices, the effectiveness of vaccinations, early illness warning indicators, and the functions of modern medicine, research, and therapy.

What You Should Remember

- As a vigilant protector of your body against illnesses and outside threats, your immune system is an outstanding defense system.

- The place you live and your decisions can either strengthen or damage your immune system.

- A robust and resilient immune system is possible by lifestyle choices such as stress management, sleep, exercise, and nutrition.

- Knowing the science underlying vaccines is essential to making intelligent choices, as vaccinations are a potent tool in the fight against many infectious diseases.

- Maintaining good health requires recognizing early warning symptoms of illness, understanding when to seek medical assistance, and using efficient home remedies.

- Although they have drawbacks, medical interventions like antibiotics, antivirals, and antifungals provide strong immune system support.

- Modern science in genetic engineering, personalized medicine, and immunotherapy is transforming healthcare and promises extremely individualized, efficient treatments.

A Knowledgeable and Proactive Approach to Health

When it comes to improving your health, your greatest weapon is knowledge. You now possess the knowledge and understanding required to make wise choices regarding your health. The components of a robust immune system, early sickness warning indicators, and the variety of resources available, from immunizations to state-of-the-art treatments—have all been covered. However, knowledge alone is insufficient. Your ability to apply this knowledge to your life gives you empowerment. Making decisions that promote your health is crucial, whether those decisions are related to daily routines, vaccine choices, or working with medical specialists.

Take Charge of Your Well-Being

You are the keeper of your health, which is a priceless asset. It is my aim that this book has motivated you to take control of your health and to actively engage in the continuous process of living a better, more fulfilling life. Instead of being a mystery force, your immune system is a flexible, dynamic barrier that changes depending on your decisions. You can boost your immune system, protect yourself from illness, and live a better quality of life by accepting the knowledge you've received and acting proactively.

Remember that maintaining your health is a lifetime journey, and you have the ability to write your own narrative and be the protagonist, provided you have the appropriate resources and attitude. As your loyal companion, your immune system can help you live a vibrant, resilient, and well-being-filled existence if you know how to support and understand it.

WORDS	MEANING
Pathogen	An organism, such as bacteria, that causes sickness
Virus	Infecting a living cell with a nonliving particle that contains protein and DNA/RNA
Antigen	Substance that elicits an immunological reaction
Innate immune system	non-specific defense mechanism
Adaptive immune system	Antigen-specific defense mechanism
B cells	Immunological memory-supporting white blood cells that manufacture antibodies

WORDS	MEANING
T cells	White blood cells with specific functions to support B cells (helper T) and to actively destroy diseased cells (killer T)
Vaccine	An inoculated pathogen that has been destroyed or rendered weaker and that generates immunity
Antibody	Specialized protein with a Y structure that tags antigens for degradation
Cell-mediated Immunity	Immunological response that is adaptive, in which T cells eliminate foreign cells
Humoral immunity	Immune response that is adaptive and dependent on antibody activity

www.ingramcontent.com/pod-product-compliance
Lightning Source LLC
Chambersburg PA
CBHW070913260726
48661CB00004B/1717